The Healthy Gut Diet Book

Fill Your Stomach, Improve Your Health: An All-Inclusive Handbook for a Gut-Healthy Diet

Thelma Howard

Copyright
© 2024 by [Thelma Howard]

All rights reserved. No part of this publication may be reproduced, distributed, or transmitted in any form or by any means, including photocopying, recording, or other electronic or mechanical methods, without the prior written permission of the publisher, except in the case of brief quotations embodied in critical reviews and certain other noncommercial uses permitted by copyright law.

This book is intended for informational purposes only and is not a substitute for professional medical advice, diagnosis, or treatment. The author and publisher disclaim any liability for the decisions you make based on the information provided. Consult with a qualified healthcare professional for personalized advice regarding your health and well-being.

Table of Contents

INTRODUCTION

In the realm of wellness and nutrition, embark on a journey with "The Healthy Gut Diet Book." As the sun rises over a bustling city, a protagonist emerges – not a person, but the often-overlooked hero within each of us: the gut. This book unveils the extraordinary world of gut health, a cornerstone of overall well-being.

Picture a bustling marketplace where the body's internal functions exchange goods and services. Amidst the hustle, the gut plays a vital role, acting as the chief negotiator for nutrient absorption, immune defense, and metabolic harmony. Yet, this unsung hero faces adversaries in the form of processed foods, stress, and sedentary lifestyles.

Our narrative unfolds with a mission: to empower readers with the knowledge and tools to cultivate a resilient and thriving gut. Through engaging chapters, we navigate the labyrinth of digestive intricacies, demystify misconceptions, and introduce the art of crafting a nourishing, gut-centric diet.

With a blend of science and practicality, this book is not just a guide but a companion on the quest for holistic well-being. The recipes, meal plans, and insights within these pages form a roadmap, guiding readers toward a healthier, happier life through the gateway of a vibrant gut. Join us in this narrative of wellness, where the gut takes center stage, and the journey to a healthier you begins.

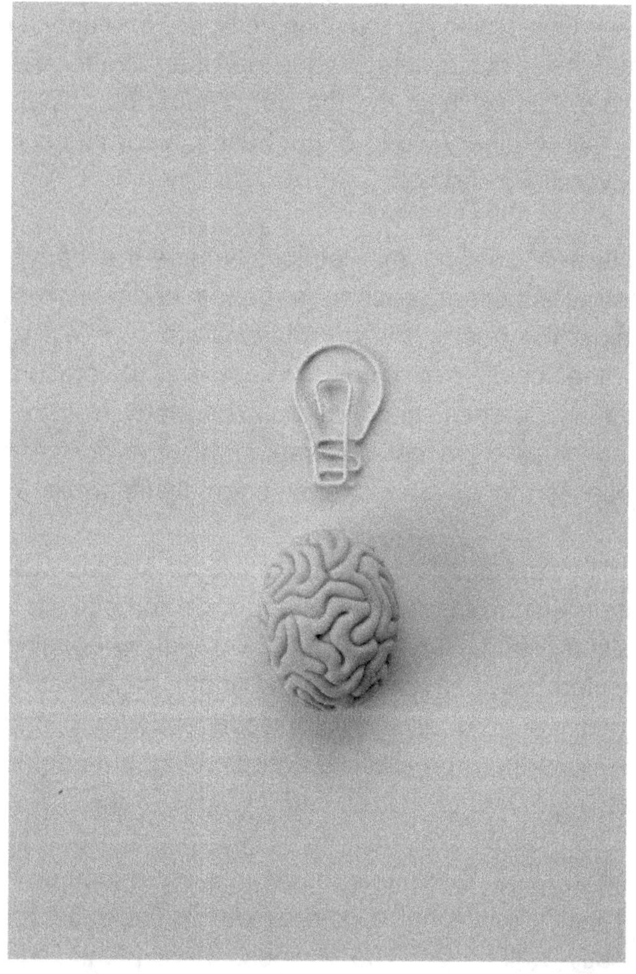

CHAPTER ONE

Understanding the Gut

A Brief Overview

"Understanding the Gut: A Brief Overview" serves as a foundational chapter in our exploration of the healthy gut diet. Delving into the intricate world of the gastrointestinal system, this section provides a concise yet comprehensive insight into the pivotal role the gut plays in our overall well-being.

The gut, often referred to as the gastrointestinal tract, is a marvel of biological engineering. Comprising the stomach, small intestine, and large intestine, it serves as the primary organ for digestion and nutrient absorption. Beyond its digestive functions, the gut houses a complex ecosystem of microorganisms known as the gut microbiota. This diverse community of bacteria, viruses, and fungi plays a crucial role in maintaining a balanced and functional digestive system.

Our overview elucidates the gut's multifaceted responsibilities, from breaking down food into absorbable nutrients to facilitating immune responses. It explores the intricate web of neural and hormonal communication between the gut and the brain, emphasizing the gut-brain axis and its impact on mood and cognitive functions.

Additionally, we touch upon the gut's role in metabolism, energy regulation, and waste elimination. Understanding the gut's dynamic interplay with various bodily systems is fundamental to appreciating its significance in fostering overall health.

In this brief yet informative chapter, readers will gain a solid foundation for the subsequent exploration of the healthy gut diet. From the anatomical intricacies to the symbiotic relationships within the gut microbiome, "Understanding the Gut" sets the stage for a deeper comprehension of the profound impact a well-nourished gut can have on one's health and vitality.

Importance of the Gut Health

The "Importance of Gut Health" is a pivotal theme in our exploration of wellness, as the gut serves as a central orchestrator of various physiological processes crucial for overall health. This chapter elucidates the profound impact that a well-maintained gut can have on an individual's physical and mental well-being.

At its core, a healthy gut is synonymous with a balanced and diverse gut microbiota, a community of trillions of microorganisms residing within the gastrointestinal tract. The symbiotic relationship between the host and these microbes influences digestion, nutrient absorption, and immune system modulation. The gut microbiota also plays a vital role in protecting against harmful pathogens, bolstering the body's defense mechanisms.

Moreover, the chapter delves into the intricate connection between gut health and mental well-being. The gut-brain axis, a bidirectional communication network between the gut and the central nervous system, highlights the impact of gut health on mood, cognitive functions, and even conditions like anxiety and depression. Understanding this connection underscores the importance of nurturing a healthy gut for mental resilience.

The significance of gut health extends to metabolic processes, with implications for weight management and energy regulation. A well-functioning gut contributes to efficient nutrient utilization and aids in maintaining a healthy body weight.

Ultimately, this chapter serves as a compelling motivator for individuals to prioritize their gut health, recognizing it not only as a cornerstone of digestive vitality but as a key influencer of holistic well-being.

Key Components of a Healthy Gut Diet

"Key Components of a Healthy Gut Diet" forms the essence of our journey toward optimal gut health, shedding light on the dietary elements crucial for fostering a resilient and thriving gastrointestinal system. This section is a comprehensive guide, breaking down the essential components that contribute to a nourishing and gut-friendly diet.

1. Probiotic-rich Foods
    - Explores the importance of incorporating probiotics, beneficial bacteria, into the diet.
   - Highlights fermented foods like yogurt, kefir, sauerkraut, and kimchi as excellent sources.
    - Discusses the role of probiotics in maintaining a healthy balance within the gut microbiota.

2. Fiber and Gut Health
   - Emphasizes the significance of dietary fiber in promoting digestive regularity.
   - Explores various high-fiber foods, including fruits, vegetables, whole grains, and legumes.
    - Discusses how fiber acts as a prebiotic, nourishing the gut microbiota and supporting its diversity.

3. Nutrient-Rich Choices

        - Addresses the importance of a well-rounded, nutrient-dense diet for overall health.

    - Highlights key vitamins and minerals that contribute to gut function, such as vitamin A, C, D, and zinc.

    - Encourages the inclusion of a variety of colorful fruits and vegetables for their diverse nutritional profiles.

Understanding these key components involves recognizing the synergy between them and their collective impact on gut health. The chapter provides practical tips for incorporating these elements into everyday meals, empowering readers to make informed dietary choices that prioritize the well-being of their digestive system.

By focusing on probiotics, fiber, and nutrient-rich foods, individuals can proactively support their gut health, laying the foundation for enhanced digestion, improved immune function, and a host of other benefits that contribute to overall vitality. This section serves as a roadmap for crafting a diet that not only nourishes the body but also nurtures the intricate ecosystem within the gut.

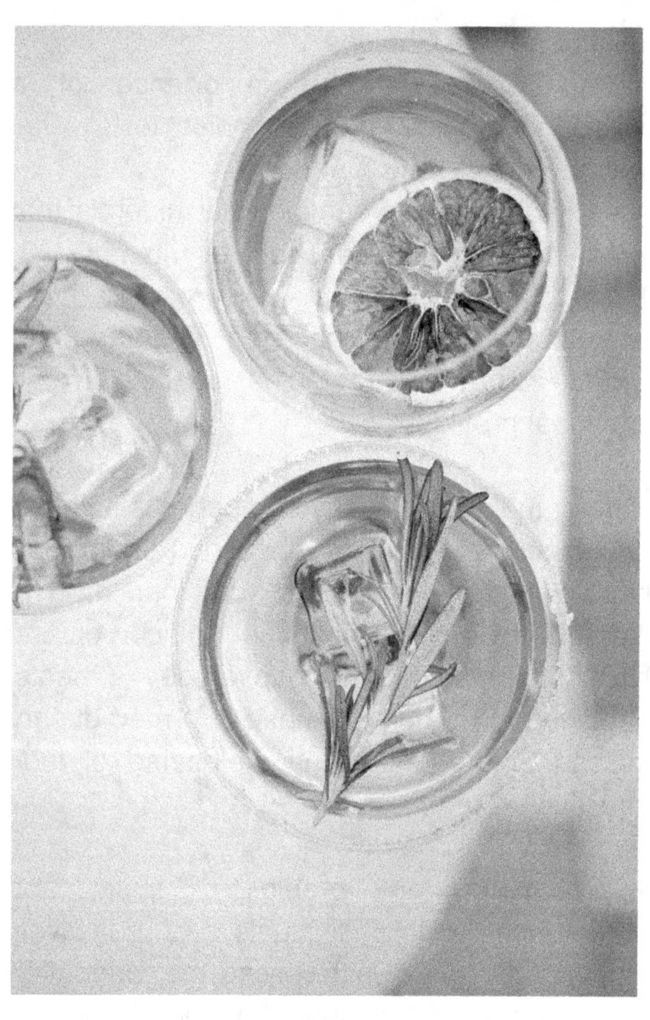

CHAPTER TWO

Gut-Friendly Recipes 01

"Gut-Friendly Recipes" opens a world of culinary exploration designed to promote digestive health and well-being. This section of our book provides a diverse array of delicious and nutritious recipes, carefully curated to support and nourish the gut microbiota while satisfying the palate.

Breakfast Ideas

Embarking on a day with gut-friendly breakfast options sets a positive tone not just for the morning but for overall well-being. This comprehensive guide explores the principles and benefits of incorporating gut-friendly choices into your breakfast routine, providing a foundation for a vibrant and energized day.

1. Probiotic-Rich Yogurt Parfait

- Begin the day with a bowl of plain Greek yogurt, a potent source of probiotics beneficial for gut health. Probiotics promote a balanced gut microbiome, aiding digestion and bolstering the immune system.

- Layer the yogurt with fresh berries, rich in antioxidants, and top with a sprinkle of chia seeds for added fiber and omega-3 fatty acids.

2. **Fiber-Focused Whole Grain Oatmeal**

   - Opt for whole grain oats as a fiber-rich foundation for your breakfast. Fiber supports digestive regularity and promotes a sense of fullness, preventing mid-morning energy crashes.

   - Enhance your oatmeal with sliced bananas for potassium, a vital nutrient for heart health, and a dollop of almond butter for healthy fats.

3. **Colorful Veggie Omelette**

   - Include a rainbow of vegetables in your morning omelette. Bell peppers, spinach, tomatoes, and mushrooms not only provide a variety of essential nutrients but also contribute to a diverse gut microbiome.

   - Cook your omelette with olive oil, an excellent source of monounsaturated fats that support heart health.

4. **Fermented Foods Fiesta**

   - Experiment with fermented foods like kimchi or sauerkraut to add a tangy kick to your breakfast. These foods are teeming with probiotics, promoting gut microbial diversity.

- Serve alongside whole grain toast topped with avocado for a nutrient-dense and satisfying meal.

5. **Smoothie Bliss with Greens**
   - Craft a nutrient-packed smoothie by blending leafy greens like kale or spinach with fruits, such as berries and a banana. The combination provides a mix of vitamins, antioxidants, and fiber.
   - Enhance the smoothie with a spoonful of yogurt for probiotics and chia seeds for an omega-3 boost.

By incorporating these gut-friendly breakfast options, you not only nourish your body with essential nutrients but also actively support the health of your gut. These choices promote a balanced and thriving gut microbiome, contributing to improved digestion, enhanced nutrient absorption, and overall vitality. Starting your day with these positive and nutritious options creates a ripple effect, influencing your energy levels and well-being throughout the day.

Gut-friendly Breakfast Recipes

Embarking on a day with gut-friendly breakfasts is a delightful and health-conscious choice. This section of our book not only introduces a variety of nutritious morning options but also provides step-by-step guidance on how to prepare these gut-loving meals.

1. **Probiotic-Packed Smoothie Bowl**
   - Ingredients:
     - 1 cup plain Greek yogurt (probiotic-rich)
     - Mixed berries (antioxidant boost)
     - Banana slices (potassium)
     - Chia seeds (fiber and omega-3 fatty acids)
   - Preparation:
     - Blend the yogurt and half of the mixed berries until smooth.
     - Pour the smoothie into a bowl and top it with the remaining berries, banana slices, and a sprinkle of chia seeds.

2. **Overnight Oats with Kefir**
   - Ingredients:
     - 1/2 cup rolled oats (fiber)
     - 1/2 cup kefir (probiotic-rich)
     - 1 tablespoon honey (optional)
     - Sliced almonds (nutrient-rich)
   - Preparation:

- Mix oats and kefir in a jar, cover, and refrigerate overnight.

- In the morning, stir well, add honey if desired, and top with sliced almonds for added crunch.

3. **Fiber-Focused Avocado Toast**
   - Ingredients:
     - Whole-grain bread (fiber)
     - Avocado slices (healthy fats)
     - Cherry tomatoes (antioxidants)
     - Sprinkle of flaxseeds (omega-3 fatty acids)
   - Preparation:
     - Toast the bread and spread avocado slices on top.
     - Arrange cherry tomatoes and sprinkle flaxseeds for an extra nutritional boost.

4. **Yogurt Parfait with Nuts and Seeds**
   - Ingredients:
     - Low-fat yogurt (probiotic-rich)
     - Granola (fiber)
     - Mixed nuts (omega-3 fatty acids)
     - Fresh fruit slices (vitamins and antioxidants)
   - Preparation:
     - Layer yogurt, granola, and mixed nuts in a glass or bowl.

- Top with fresh fruit slices for a colorful and nutrient-packed parfait.

These recipes not only cater to the nutritional needs of the gut but also showcase the versatility and deliciousness of gut-friendly breakfasts. By incorporating probiotic-rich ingredients, fiber, and nutrient-dense foods, these morning delights set the stage for a day of sustained energy and digestive well-being. The step-by-step instructions make these recipes accessible for individuals looking to kickstart their mornings with a boost to gut health.

The importance of incorporating diverse nutrients to kickstart the morning.

The importance of incorporating diverse nutrients to kickstart the morning cannot be overstated as it lays the foundation for sustained energy, cognitive function, and overall well-being throughout the day. A breakfast rich in diverse nutrients not only fuels the body but also contributes to a balanced and thriving gut, reinforcing the symbiotic relationship between nutrition and gut health.

1. **Energy Boost**
- A breakfast that includes a variety of nutrients provides a balanced source of energy.

Carbohydrates from whole grains, proteins from sources like yogurt or eggs, and healthy fats from avocados or nuts work together to offer a sustained release of energy, preventing mid-morning slumps.

2. **Cognitive Function**
  - Diverse nutrients play a crucial role in supporting cognitive function. Foods rich in omega-3 fatty acids, such as chia seeds or fatty fish, contribute to brain health. Antioxidant-packed fruits and vegetables protect against oxidative stress, promoting mental clarity and focus.

3. **Blood Sugar Regulation**
  - Including a mix of carbohydrates, proteins, and fats in breakfast helps regulate blood sugar levels. This balance prevents rapid spikes and crashes in blood sugar, promoting stable energy levels and reducing the risk of cravings later in the day.

4. **Gut Microbiome Health**
  - A diverse range of nutrients supports the health of the gut microbiome. Fiber from whole grains and fruits acts as a prebiotic, nourishing beneficial bacteria in the gut. Probiotics from yogurt or fermented foods further enhance

microbial diversity, contributing to optimal gut function.

5. **Nutrient Absorption**

- Breakfast sets the stage for nutrient absorption throughout the day. Including a variety of nutrients ensures that the body receives a broad spectrum of essential vitamins and minerals, supporting various bodily functions, from immune health to bone strength.

6. **Mood Regulation**

- Nutrient-rich breakfasts can positively impact mood. Foods containing amino acids, such as those found in eggs or lean meats, contribute to the synthesis of neurotransmitters like serotonin, promoting a sense of well-being and positivity.

7. **Weight Management**

- Diverse nutrients play a role in satiety, helping control appetite and prevent overeating later in the day. A well-balanced breakfast can contribute to weight management by providing the body with the necessary nutrients without excess calories.

Incorporating diverse nutrients into the morning routine is a holistic approach to nutrition that goes beyond simply satisfying hunger. It is an investment in overall health, setting the stage for improved energy, cognitive function, and a resilient gut. As individuals prioritize a diverse and nutritious breakfast, they pave the way for a day filled with vitality and well-being.

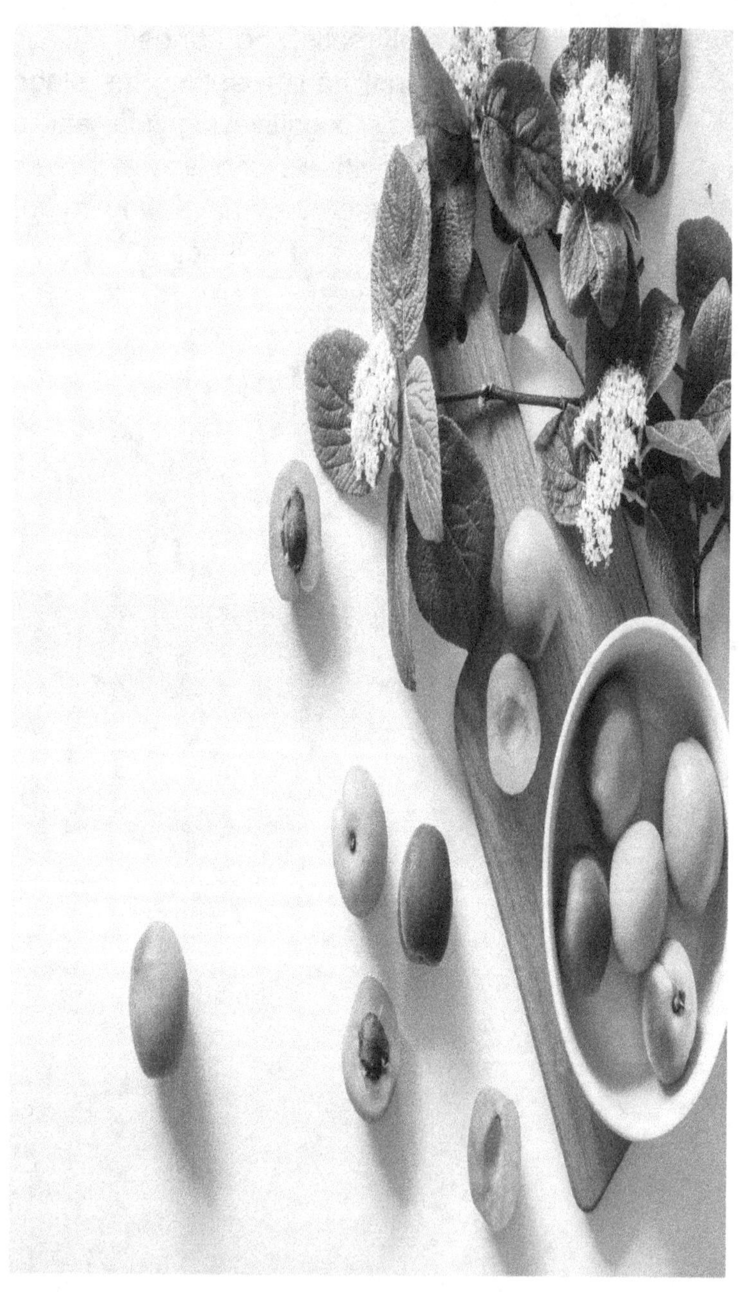

CHAPTER THREE

Gut-Friendly Recipes 02

Lunch and Dinner Recipes

Savory Options that Blend Flavor with Gut-Friendly Ingredients" present an exciting array of dishes designed to tantalize taste buds while promoting digestive health. This comprehensive guide introduces flavorful recipes crafted with ingredients that support a balanced and thriving gut, ensuring that every meal is a delicious and nutritious experience.

1. Fermented Vegetable Stir-Fry

- This vibrant stir-fry combines a medley of colorful vegetables with the tangy goodness of fermented foods like kimchi or sauerkraut.

- Sautee bell peppers, broccoli, and carrots in olive oil, adding fermented vegetables for a probiotic kick.

- Serve over quinoa or brown rice for a fiber-rich and nutrient-packed meal.

2. Grilled Fish Tacos with Cabbage Slaw

- Grilled fish tacos offer a delightful combination of lean protein and vibrant flavors.

- Marinate white fish fillets with lime juice, garlic, and cumin before grilling.
- Assemble the tacos with a crunchy cabbage slaw, rich in fiber, and top with a dollop of yogurt for added probiotics.

3. Quinoa Bowls with Roasted Vegetables
- Quinoa serves as a versatile base for a nutrient-dense bowl filled with roasted vegetables.
- Roast sweet potatoes, Brussels sprouts, and cherry tomatoes with olive oil and herbs.
- Combine with cooked quinoa and drizzle with a lemon-tahini dressing for a satisfying and gut-friendly meal.

4. Chickpea and Spinach Curry
- This plant-based curry combines the protein punch of chickpeas with the nutrient richness of spinach.
- Simmer chickpeas and spinach in a flavorful curry sauce made with turmeric, cumin, and coriander.
- Serve over brown rice or quinoa for a fiber-packed and gut-loving dinner option.

5. Miso-Glazed Salmon with Asparagus

- Miso-glazed salmon provides a savory umami flavor while delivering heart-healthy omega-3 fatty acids.
- Roast asparagus with olive oil and serve alongside miso-glazed salmon for a delicious and nutrient-rich dinner.
- Miso, a fermented soy product, adds an extra layer of gut-friendly benefits.

6. Mushroom and Lentil Stuffed Peppers
- Stuffed peppers offer a creative way to combine protein-packed lentils with earthy mushrooms.
- Cook lentils and mushrooms with herbs and spices before stuffing into bell peppers.
- Bake until tender and serve with a side of leafy greens for added fiber.

These savory lunch and dinner recipes not only satisfy the palate but also prioritize gut health through a thoughtful selection of ingredients. By incorporating probiotic-rich foods, lean proteins, and a variety of vegetables, these dishes make each meal a delightful and nourishing experience. Experimenting with these recipes ensures a diverse and gut-friendly approach to lunch and dinner, contributing to overall digestive well-being.

Feature Dishes

Fermented Vegetable Stir-Fry
Ingredients
- Mixed vegetables (bell peppers, broccoli, carrots)
- Fermented vegetables (kimchi or sauerkraut)
- Olive oil
- Soy sauce
- Garlic and ginger (minced)
- Brown rice or quinoa (optional, for serving)

Preparation
1. Heat olive oil in a pan over medium heat.
2. Add the ginger and garlic, minced, and sauté until aromatic.
3. Stir in mixed vegetables, cooking until slightly tender yet crisp.
4. Incorporate fermented vegetables, adding a unique tangy flavor and probiotic benefits.
5. Drizzle with soy sauce for a savory finish.
6. Serve over a bed of quinoa or brown rice for a complete, fiber-rich meal.

Grilled Fish Tacos with Cabbage Slaw
Ingredients
- White fish fillets (tilapia, cod)
- Corn or whole wheat tortillas
- Cabbage (shredded)

- Greek yogurt (plain, for slaw)
- Lime juice
- Cumin, garlic powder, paprika
- Avocado slices (optional)

Preparation
1. Marinate fish fillets in lime juice, cumin, garlic powder, and paprika.
2. Grill the fish until cooked through and slightly charred.
3. In a bowl, mix shredded cabbage with Greek yogurt, lime juice, and a pinch of salt for the slaw.
4. Warm tortillas and assemble tacos with grilled fish, cabbage slaw, and optional avocado slices.
5. Garnish with fresh cilantro and an extra squeeze of lime.

Quinoa Bowls with Roasted Vegetables
Ingredients
- Quinoa
- Sweet potatoes (cubed)
- Brussels sprouts (halved)
- Cherry tomatoes
- Olive oil, salt, pepper
- Lemon-tahini dressing

Preparation

1. Cook quinoa according to package instructions.
2. Toss sweet potatoes, Brussels sprouts, and cherry tomatoes in olive oil, salt, and pepper.
3. Roast vegetables in the oven until caramelized and tender.
4. Combine cooked quinoa with the roasted vegetables.
5. Drizzle with a lemon-tahini dressing for a burst of flavor and creaminess.
6. Top with fresh herbs or feta cheese for added appeal.

These featured dishes offer a spectrum of flavors, textures, and nutritional benefits. The fermented vegetable stir-fry introduces probiotics into the meal, promoting gut health. Grilled fish tacos combine lean protein with a crunchy cabbage slaw for a satisfying and nutritious option. Quinoa bowls with roasted vegetables provide a colorful and nutrient-packed experience, with the lemon-tahini dressing adding a zesty twist. Experimenting with these recipes not only enhances your culinary skills but also contributes to a diverse and gut-friendly approach to your meals.

The benefits of lean proteins, whole grains, and plant-based foods in promoting gut health

Lean Proteins

1. Amino Acid Diversity

   - Lean proteins, such as poultry, fish, and legumes, provide a rich array of essential amino acids.

   - Amino acids are building blocks for proteins, supporting the repair and maintenance of gut tissues.

2. Collagen Formation

   - Certain lean proteins, like chicken and fish, contain collagen, supporting the integrity of the intestinal lining.

   - Collagen helps prevent the development of "leaky gut" by maintaining a strong barrier function.

3. Anti-Inflammatory Properties

   - Lean proteins often have anti-inflammatory effects, reducing the risk of chronic inflammation in the gut.

   - Chronic inflammation is associated with various digestive disorders, and incorporating lean proteins can help mitigate this risk.

4. Satiety and Weight Management

   - Proteins contribute to a feeling of fullness, aiding in weight management by reducing overall calorie intake.

   - Maintaining a healthy weight is linked to improved gut health and a lower risk of gastrointestinal issues.

Whole Grains

1. Fiber for Gut Microbiota

   - Whole grains, such as brown rice, quinoa, and oats, are excellent sources of dietary fiber.

   - Fiber acts as a prebiotic, promoting the growth of beneficial gut bacteria and enhancing microbial diversity.

2. Regulating Bowel Movements

   - Whole grains contain insoluble fiber, which gives stool more volume and promotes regular bowel motions. This promotes a healthy digestive tract and aids in the prevention of constipation.

3. Short-Chain Fatty Acids (SCFAs)

   - Fermentation of fiber in whole grains produces short-chain fatty acids (SCFAs) in the gut.

   - SCFAs play a vital role in nourishing the gut lining and regulating immune responses.

4. **Blood Sugar Regulation**

- The complex carbohydrates in whole grains provide a steady release of energy, helping to regulate blood sugar levels.

- Stable blood sugar levels contribute to overall gut health and reduce the risk of insulin-related issues.

Plant-Based Foods

1. Diverse Nutrient Profile

- Plant-based foods, including fruits, vegetables, nuts, and seeds, offer a broad spectrum of vitamins, minerals, and antioxidants.

- These nutrients support various aspects of gut health, from tissue repair to immune function.

2. Fiber and Gut Microbiome

- Plant-based diets are typically high in fiber, promoting a healthy gut microbiome.

- Fiber-rich plant foods act as substrates for beneficial bacteria, fostering a balanced and diverse microbial community.

3. Anti-Inflammatory Properties
    - Many plant-based foods possess anti-inflammatory properties, reducing inflammation in the gut.
    - This can contribute to the prevention of inflammatory bowel diseases and other digestive disorders.

4. Phytonutrients and Antioxidants
    - Phytonutrients and antioxidants in plant-based foods protect the gut from oxidative stress and inflammation.
    - These compounds support cellular health and contribute to a resilient digestive system.

Incorporating lean proteins, whole grains, and plant-based foods into your diet fosters a holistic approach to gut health. The combination of amino acids, fiber, and diverse nutrients from these sources supports digestive function, microbiome diversity, and overall well-being. As part of a balanced and varied diet, these food groups contribute to the optimal functioning of the gut and help prevent various gastrointestinal issues.

CHAPTER FOUR

Gut-Friendly Recipes 03

Snack Options

Provides satisfying and convenient snacks that contribute to gut well-being.

Greek Yogurt with Berries and Nuts

1. Probiotic Boost

   - Probiotic-rich Greek yogurt helps maintain a healthy balance of gut flora.

   - Probiotics contribute to optimal digestion and support immune function.

2. Antioxidant-Rich Berries

   - Berries, such as blueberries and strawberries, provide antioxidants that protect the gut from oxidative stress.

   - Antioxidants play a role in reducing inflammation and supporting overall gut health.

3. Omega-3 Fatty Acids from Nuts

   - Nuts, like almonds or walnuts, add a crunchy texture and provide omega-3 fatty acids.

   - Omega-3s contribute to a healthy gut lining and have anti-inflammatory effects.

4. Satisfying and Nutrient-Dense

- This snack is not only delicious but also satiating, helping to curb hunger between meals.

- The combination of protein, fiber, and healthy fats supports overall well-being.

Hummus with Raw Vegetables

1. Fiber-Rich and Digestive Support

- Hummus, made from chickpeas, is a good source of fiber that supports digestive health.

- Fiber aids in regular bowel movements and contributes to a thriving gut microbiome.

2. Colorful Raw Vegetables

- Pairing hummus with raw vegetables like carrot sticks, cucumber, and bell pepper provides a diverse array of nutrients.

- Different-colored vegetables offer various vitamins, minerals, and antioxidants.

3. Prebiotics in Vegetables

- Raw vegetables contain prebiotics that nourish beneficial gut bacteria.

- The combination of hummus and raw veggies promotes microbial diversity.

4. Quick and Convenient

- This snack requires minimal preparation, making it a convenient option for a busy day.

- It's a satisfying choice that contributes to gut health without compromising on taste.

Fermented Pickles

1. Natural Probiotics

- Fermented pickles are rich in natural probiotics due to the fermentation process.

- Probiotics from pickles support the balance of gut bacteria and aid in digestion.

2. Low in Calories

Pickles are a guilt-free snack option because they are low in calories.

- They provide flavor without the added sugars or processed ingredients found in some snacks.

3. Sodium Regulation

- While pickles are salty, they can be a suitable snack for those with sodium concerns.

- The salt content in pickles is often lower compared to many processed snacks.

4. Crunchy and Tangy

- The crunchiness and tangy flavor of fermented pickles make them a satisfying and enjoyable snack.

- They add variety to your snacking routine while supporting gut health.

Chia Seed Pudding

1. Omega-3 Fatty Acids from Chia Seeds

- Chia seeds are a rich source of omega-3 fatty acids, supporting gut and heart health.

- Omega-3s have anti-inflammatory properties, contributing to a healthy digestive system.

2. Fiber for Satiety

- Chia seeds absorb liquid and form a gel-like consistency, providing a satisfying texture.

- The fiber content in chia seeds supports satiety and digestive regularity.

3. Customizable and Tasty

- Chia seed pudding is highly customizable with various flavor options such as vanilla, chocolate, or fruity variations.

- It offers a sweet treat without the refined sugars often found in traditional desserts.

4. Preparation in Advance

- Chia seed pudding can be prepared in advance, making it a convenient grab-and-go snack.

- It's a nutrient-dense option that contributes to gut well-being in a delicious manner.

Incorporating these satisfying and convenient snacks into your routine not only curbs hunger but also actively supports gut health. The combination of probiotics, fiber, and nutrient-rich ingredients makes these snacks not just delicious treats but integral components of a holistic approach to well-being.

Recipes for probiotic-rich snacks.

Homemade Yogurt with Nuts and Seeds
Ingredients
- 2 cups whole milk
- 2 tablespoons plain yogurt with live cultures (as a starter)
- Mixed nuts (almonds, walnuts) and seeds (chia seeds, flaxseeds)
- Honey or maple syrup for sweetness (optional)

Preparation

1. Heat the milk in a saucepan until it reaches around 180°F (82°C), then let it cool to around 110°F (43°C).
2. In a bowl, mix the plain yogurt with a small amount of the warm milk to create a smooth mixture.
3. Add the yogurt mixture back into the warm milk and stir well.
4. Cover the mixture and let it sit undisturbed in a warm place for 6-12 hours, allowing it to ferment into yogurt.
5. Once set, refrigerate the yogurt.
6. Serve the homemade yogurt with a sprinkle of mixed nuts and seeds. **If desired, drizzle with maple syrup or honey.**

Fermented Pickles
Ingredients
- 1 pound small cucumbers
- 2 cups water
- 1 1/2 tablespoons salt
- Fresh dill
- Garlic cloves
- Peppercorns
- Optional: mustard seeds, coriander seeds, red pepper flakes

Preparation

1. Wash the cucumbers thoroughly and cut off the blossom end.

2. In a jar, combine water and salt to create a brine.

3. Add fresh dill, garlic cloves, peppercorns, and any optional spices to the jar.

4. Pack the cucumbers into the jar tightly.

5. Pour the brine over the cucumbers, ensuring they are fully submerged.

6. Close the jar and let it sit at room temperature for about 3-7 days, depending on your preference for pickle intensity.

7. Once fermented, refrigerate the pickles.

Hummus with Raw Vegetables

Ingredients

- One can (15 ounces) of rinsed and drained chickpeas
- 1/4 cup tahini
- 1/4 cup olive oil
- 1 garlic clove, minced
- Juice of 1 lemon
- Salt and pepper to taste
- Raw vegetables (carrot sticks, cucumber slices, bell pepper strips)

Preparation
1. . In a food processor, add chickpeas, tahini, olive oil, minced garlic, and lemon juice.
2. Process until smooth, adding water if needed for desired consistency.
3. To taste, add salt and pepper for seasoning.
4. Transfer hummus to a bowl and serve with raw vegetables.

These probiotic-rich snacks not only satisfy your taste buds but also actively contribute to gut health. Homemade yogurt provides live cultures, fermented pickles introduce natural probiotics, and hummus with raw vegetables offers a fiber-packed treat. Incorporating these snacks into your routine ensures a tasty and nutritious way to support your digestive well-being.

Understanding Mindful Snacking

1. Conscious Choices
   - Mindful snacking involves making intentional and conscious choices about what and how much you eat between meals.
   - It encourages awareness of hunger cues, emotional triggers, and the nutritional value of snacks.

2. Listening to Hunger Signals

- Mindful snacking emphasizes tuning into your body's hunger signals.

- Before snacking, take a moment to assess whether you are genuinely hungry or responding to other cues like stress or boredom.

3. Balancing Macronutrients

- Choose snacks that include a balance of macronutrients – proteins, fats, and carbohydrates.

- This balance helps maintain steady energy levels and prevents quick spikes and crashes.

4. Portion Control

Pay attention to portion proportions to prevent overindulging without thinking.

- Use small bowls or plates and savor each bite to enhance satisfaction.

5. Mindful Eating Practices

- Engage in mindful eating practices during snacks, such as chewing slowly and paying attention to flavors and textures.

- This fosters a deeper connection with your food and promotes satiety.

Nutrient-Dense Snack Options

1. Protein-Packed Choices
   - Incorporate protein-rich snacks like Greek yogurt, lean meats, or nuts.
   - Protein helps keep you feeling full and supports muscle maintenance and repair.
2. Fiber-Rich Options
   - Choose snacks high in fiber, such as fruits, vegetables, and whole grains.
   - Fiber contributes to digestive health and provides a sustained release of energy.

3. Healthy Fats
   - Include snacks with healthy fats, like avocados, nuts, or seeds.
   - Healthy fats contribute to satiety and provide a concentrated source of energy.
4. Hydration
   - **Drink plenty of water throughout the day since often people confuse thirst for hunger.**
   - Water or herbal teas can be excellent choices for mindful hydration.

Mindful Snack Ideas

1. Apple Slices with Nut Butter
   - Pairing apple slices with nut butter provides a combination of fiber, natural sugars, and healthy fats.

2. Yogurt Parfait
   - Layering yogurt with granola and fresh berries creates a satisfying and nutrient-dense snack.

3. Vegetable Sticks with Hummus
   - Raw vegetable sticks with hummus offer a crunchy, fiber-rich option with a balance of proteins and healthy fats.

4. Trail Mix
   - Create a custom trail mix with a variety of nuts, seeds, and dried fruits.
   - **Keep an eye on serving sizes to limit your consumption of calories.**

5. Dark Chocolate with Almonds
   - A small serving of dark chocolate paired with almonds combines antioxidants with healthy fats and protein.

Creating a Mindful Snacking Environment
1. Limit Distractions
   - Avoid snacking while distracted by screens or work.
   - Create a calm environment to enhance the mindful eating experience.

2. Savoring the Moment
   - Take a moment to appreciate the flavors, textures, and aromas of your snack.
   - Mindful snacking is about enjoying the experience of eating.

3. Respecting Cravings
   - Acknowledge and respect your cravings without judgment.
   - Choose snacks that satisfy your cravings in a balanced and mindful way.

By incorporating mindful snacking into your daily routine, you not only maintain steady energy levels but also cultivate a healthier relationship with food. It's a practice that encourages conscious choices, fosters a connection with your body's signals, and promotes overall well-being.

CHAPTER FIVE

Understanding the Significance of Meal Planning for Gut Health

1. Consistency and Routine

- Meal planning establishes a regular eating routine, which is beneficial for gut health.

- Consistent mealtimes help regulate digestive processes and support the circadian rhythm.

2. Balanced Nutrition

- Planning meals in advance allows for intentional inclusion of a variety of nutrients.

- A well-balanced diet ensures that the gut receives the necessary components for optimal functioning.

3. Supporting the Gut Microbiome

- Incorporating a diverse range of foods in meal planning promotes microbial diversity in the gut.

- Different types of fibers, prebiotics, and probiotics contribute to a thriving gut microbiome.

4. Minimizing Processed Foods

- Thoughtful meal planning reduces reliance on processed and convenience foods.

- Processed foods often contain additives that may negatively impact gut health, while whole foods provide essential nutrients.

Key Components of Gut-Healthy Meal Planning

1. Variety of Colorful Vegetables

- Plan meals that include a rainbow of vegetables, providing a range of vitamins, minerals, and antioxidants.

- Different vegetables support different aspects of gut health and contribute to microbial diversity.

2. High-Fiber Foods

- Include high-fiber foods like whole grains, legumes, fruits, and vegetables in your meal plans.

- Fiber promotes regular bowel movements and serves as a prebiotic, nourishing beneficial gut bacteria.

3. Lean Proteins

- Incorporate lean protein sources such as poultry, fish, beans, and tofu.

- Protein is essential for tissue repair, and lean sources support overall digestive health.

4. Fermented Foods
   - Plan for fermented foods like yogurt, kefir, sauerkraut, or kimchi.
   - These foods contain probiotics, which contribute to a balanced and resilient gut microbiome.

5. Healthy Fats
   - Incorporate foods like avocados, almonds, seeds, and olive oil that are good sources of fat.
   - Omega-3 fatty acids in particular support anti-inflammatory processes in the gut.

6. Hydration
   - Ensure adequate hydration by incorporating water, herbal teas, and other low-sugar beverages into your meal plan.
   - Digestion and nutrition absorption depend on being hydrated.

Practical Meal Planning Tips for Gut Health

1. Batch Cooking
   - Prepare larger quantities of meals during the week to have leftovers for subsequent days.
   - This reduces reliance on last-minute, potentially less nutritious food choices.

2. Prep Ahead

- Wash, chop, and portion fruits and vegetables in advance to streamline meal preparation.

- Having prepared ingredients makes it easier to incorporate them into meals throughout the week.

3. Mindful Portion Control

- Consider portion sizes to avoid overeating, which can stress the digestive system.

- Smaller, balanced meals support optimal digestion.

4. Experiment with New Recipes

- Keep meal planning interesting by trying new recipes with different ingredients.

- Variety introduces a range of nutrients and flavors, enhancing the overall dining experience.

5. Listen to Your Body

- Take note of your feelings after eating various foods.

- Adjust your meal planning based on your body's responses, considering any sensitivities or intolerances.

Long-Term Benefits of Gut-Healthy Meal Planning

1. Enhanced Digestion

- Consistent, well-balanced meals support efficient digestion and nutrient absorption.

- This contributes to overall digestive comfort and function.

2. Improved Gut Microbiome Diversity
   - A variety of gut-friendly foods fosters a diverse and resilient gut microbiome.
   - A balanced microbiome is linked to better immune function and overall health.
3. Sustained Energy Levels
   - Nutrient-dense meal planning helps maintain steady energy levels throughout the day.
   - This reduces the likelihood of energy crashes and supports sustained vitality.
4. Weight Management
   - Planning meals mindfully aids in weight management by controlling portion sizes and promoting mindful eating.
   - Maintaining a healthy weight positively influences gut health.
5. Reduced Gastrointestinal Discomfort
   - By avoiding certain triggers and incorporating gut-friendly foods, meal planning can reduce gastrointestinal discomfort.
   - It supports individuals with specific digestive conditions in managing symptoms.
6. Holistic Well-Being

- Gut-healthy meal planning is not just about digestive health but contributes to overall well-being.

- It supports immune function, mental health, and various physiological processes.

Meal planning for optimal gut health is a holistic approach that involves thoughtful consideration of food choices, regularity, and mindful eating practices. By incorporating a variety of nutrient-dense foods and cultivating healthy eating habits, individuals can promote a resilient gut and enhance their overall well-being.

CHAPTER SIX

Incorporating Lifestyle Habits for a Healthy Gut

1. Balanced Diet
   - Prioritize a well-balanced diet rich in fiber, whole grains, lean proteins, and a variety of fruits and vegetables.
   - A diverse range of nutrients supports gut health and promotes a thriving microbiome.

2. Stay Hydrated
   - **For both digestion and general health, one must drink enough water.**

   - Water helps maintain the mucosal lining of the intestines and supports the movement of food through the digestive tract.

3. Regular Physical Activity
   - Engage in regular exercise to promote a healthy gut.
   - Physical activity stimulates the contraction of intestinal muscles, aiding in the movement of food and waste through the digestive system.

4. Adequate Sleep

- Prioritize sufficient and quality sleep to support overall well-being, including gut health.

- Sleep deprivation can upset the delicate balance of gut flora and aggravate digestive problems.

5. Stress Management

- Chronic stress can negatively impact the gut and contribute to digestive problems.

- Use stress-reduction strategies including deep breathing, mindfulness, and meditation.

6. Limit Antibiotic Use

- Use antibiotics judiciously and only as prescribed by a healthcare professional.

- Excessive antibiotic use can disrupt the balance of gut bacteria, leading to dysbiosis.

7. Probiotics and Fermented Foods

- Include probiotics in your diet through supplements or naturally fermented foods like yogurt, kefir, sauerkraut, and kimchi.

- Probiotics support the proper balance of intestinal flora.

8. Limit Artificial Sweeteners
   - Artificial sweeteners may negatively impact the gut microbiome.
   - Limit the consumption of artificial sweeteners and opt for natural sweeteners in moderation.

9. Avoid Overuse of NSAIDs
   - Nonsteroidal anti-inflammatory drugs (NSAIDs) can contribute to gastrointestinal issues.
   - Use NSAIDs cautiously and under the guidance of a healthcare professional.

10. Mindful Eating
   - By being aware of your body's signals of hunger and fullness, cultivate mindful eating.

   - Chew food thoroughly to aid in digestion and nutrient absorption.

11. Prebiotics from Whole Foods
   - Include prebiotic-rich foods like garlic, onions, leeks, asparagus, and bananas in your diet.
   - Prebiotics nourish beneficial gut bacteria.

12. Maintain a Healthy Weight

- Aim for a healthy weight through a combination of balanced nutrition and regular physical activity.

- Excess weight, especially around the abdominal area, can impact gut health.

13. Limit Processed Foods

- Processed foods often contain additives and preservatives that may negatively affect gut health.

- Choose whole, minimally processed foods whenever possible.

14. Regular Health Check-ups

- Schedule regular check-ups with healthcare professionals to address any digestive concerns.

- Early detection and management of digestive issues contribute to long-term gut health.

15. Environmental Factors

- Be mindful of environmental factors that may impact gut health, such as exposure to pollutants and toxins.

- Minimize exposure where possible and support detoxification through a healthy lifestyle.

Personalized Approach to Gut Health

1. Know Your Body

  - Pay attention to how your body responds to different foods and lifestyle choices.

  - Adjust your habits based on your individual needs and sensitivities.

2. Consult with Healthcare Professionals

  - Seek guidance from healthcare professionals, including registered dietitians and gastroenterologists, for personalized advice.

  - Professional insights can help address specific gut-related concerns.

3. Gradual Changes

  - Implement changes gradually to allow your body to adapt.

  - Sudden and drastic shifts in diet or lifestyle may disrupt the balance of your gut microbiome.

4. Be Patient

  - Enhancing intestinal well-being is a steady process, and personal reactions could differ.

  - Be patient and consistent with positive lifestyle habits for long-term benefits.

By incorporating these lifestyle tips into your daily routine, you create a foundation for a healthy gut. Remember that individual responses vary, and it's essential to adopt a personalized approach based on your unique needs and preferences. A holistic commitment to overall well-being, both physically and mentally, contributes to a resilient and thriving gut.

CHAPTER SEVEN

Misconceptions about Gut Health

1. Misconception: Probiotics Cure All Digestive Issues:

   - Reality: While probiotics offer benefits, they are not a one-size-fits-all solution. The effectiveness of probiotics varies, and their impact on individual health depends on factors like the specific strains used and the person's unique microbiome.

2. Misconception: All Bacteria are Harmful:

   - Reality: The gut harbors trillions of bacteria, and not all are harmful. In fact, many bacteria are beneficial for digestion, nutrient absorption, and overall gut health. It's about maintaining a balance between beneficial and potentially harmful bacteria.

3. Misconception: Gut Health is Only About Digestion:

   -Reality: Gut health extends beyond digestion. A healthy gut contributes to overall well-being, including immune function, mental health, and even cardiovascular health. It plays a crucial role in various bodily functions beyond breaking down food.

4. Misconception: Gut Health is Static:
   -Reality: The gut microbiome is dynamic and can change over time based on factors like diet, lifestyle, and medications. It's not a fixed entity, and individuals have the ability to influence and improve their gut health through conscious choices.

5. Misconception: Probiotics Survive Indefinitely in the Gut:
   -Reality: Probiotics are living microorganisms, and their survival in the gut is influenced by various factors, including the specific strain, formulation, and individual differences. Probiotics may need continuous intake to maintain their presence in the gut.

6. Misconception: All Fiber is Equal for Gut Health:
   -Reality: Different types of fiber have varying effects on the gut. Soluble fiber, found in oats and fruits, ferments in the colon and supports beneficial bacteria. Insoluble fiber, found in wheat bran, adds bulk to stool. A diverse range of fiber sources is beneficial for gut health.

7. Misconception: Gut Issues are Solely Diet-Related:

-Reality: While diet plays a crucial role, gut health is influenced by various factors, including genetics, stress levels, sleep, physical activity, and medication use. A holistic approach is necessary to address and support overall gut well-being.

8. Misconception: Gut Health Only Affects Digestive System:

-Reality: Poor gut health can have widespread effects on the body, impacting the immune system, mental health, skin conditions, and even chronic diseases. The gut-brain axis highlights the bidirectional communication between the gut and the brain.

9. Misconception: Eliminating Gluten is Necessary for Everyone:

-Reality: While individuals with celiac disease or gluten sensitivity need to avoid gluten, it's not necessary for everyone. For many people, gluten-containing grains provide essential nutrients, and unnecessary avoidance can lead to nutritional deficiencies.

10. Misconception: Gut Health Supplements Replace a Balanced Diet:

- Reality: Supplements can complement a healthy diet, but they cannot replace the variety of nutrients obtained through whole foods. A well-rounded diet is crucial for supporting overall health, including gut health.

11. Misconception: All Digestive Discomfort Indicates a Problem:

-Reality: Occasional digestive discomfort does not necessarily indicate a chronic issue. Factors like stress, temporary dietary changes, or infections can cause short-term discomfort. **A medical expert should be consulted if symptoms are severe or persistent.**

12. Misconception: Detox Diets Always Improve Gut Health:

- Reality: Extreme detox diets may disrupt the balance of gut bacteria and lead to nutrient deficiencies. The body has its own detoxification mechanisms, and a balanced diet with fiber and hydration is generally sufficient for supporting natural detox processes.

Promoting Informed Perspectives
Understanding the nuances of gut health is essential for making informed decisions about dietary and lifestyle choices. Dispelling

common misconceptions allows individuals to approach gut health with a balanced and evidence-based mindset, ultimately contributing to overall well-being.

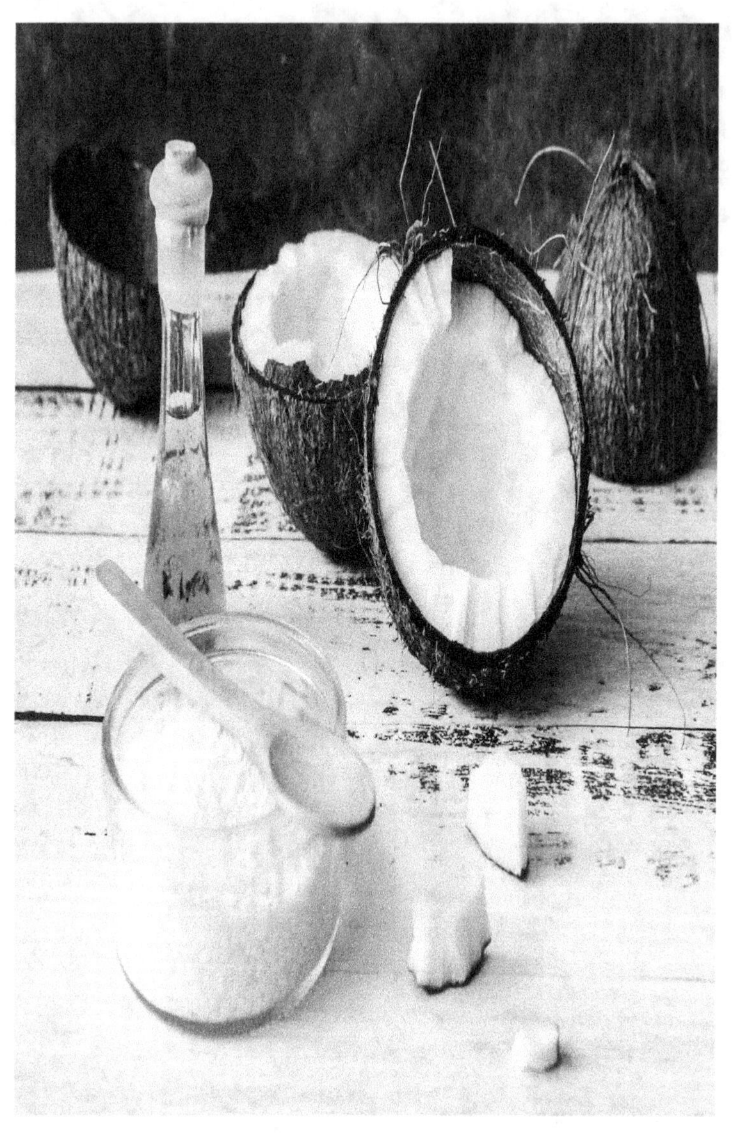

CHAPTER EIGHT

Frequently Asked Questions on Gut Health

1. What is Gut Health, and Why is it Important?

-Answer: Gut health refers to the well-being of the gastrointestinal tract and its microbiota. A healthy gut plays a crucial role in digestion, nutrient absorption, immune function, and overall well-being. It is linked to various aspects of physical and mental health.

2. How Can I Improve My Gut Health?

-Answer: Focus on a balanced diet with fiber-rich foods, lean proteins, and probiotics. Stay hydrated, manage stress, get regular exercise, and prioritize sufficient sleep. Avoid excessive use of antibiotics and processed foods. Individualized approaches may involve consulting healthcare professionals.

3. Are Probiotics Effective for Gut Health?

-Answer: Probiotics can be beneficial for gut health by promoting a balanced microbiome. However, their effectiveness varies among individuals and depends on factors like the specific strains used, dosage, and overall health. **Seeking individualised guidance from a healthcare practitioner is advised.**

4. Do I Need to Follow a Specific Diet for Gut Health?

   - Answer: A diet rich in fiber, diverse fruits and vegetables, lean proteins, and fermented foods supports gut health. There's no one-size-fits-all approach, and individual needs may vary. **If you would need individualized nutritional advice, think about speaking with a licensed dietitian.**

5. Can Gut Health Affect Mental Well-being?

   -Answer: Yes, the gut-brain connection is well-established. A healthy gut can positively impact mental health, and disruptions in gut health have been linked to conditions like anxiety and depression. Practices that support gut health often contribute to overall well-being.

6. How Long Does it Take to Improve Gut Health?

   - Answer: Improving gut health is a gradual process and varies among individuals. Changes in diet and lifestyle may show effects in a few weeks, but long-term habits are crucial for sustained improvements. Patience and consistency are key.

7. Are Gluten-Free Diets Necessary for Gut Health?

 - Answer: Gluten-free diets are essential for individuals with celiac disease or gluten sensitivity. However, for the general population, avoiding gluten may not be necessary. Gluten-containing grains provide valuable nutrients, and unnecessary elimination may lead to nutritional deficiencies.

8. Can Gut Health Affect Weight?

 -Answer: Yes, gut health can influence weight management. A balanced gut microbiome may support metabolism and contribute to maintaining a healthy weight. Factors like the diversity of gut bacteria and how they extract energy from food play a role in weight regulation.

9. Are Digestive Discomforts Normal?

 -Answer: Occasional digestive discomfort is normal and can result from various factors like diet changes, stress, or temporary infections. Persistent or severe symptoms, however, may indicate an underlying issue and should be evaluated by a healthcare professional.

10. Can Gut Health Impact Immune Function?

-Answer: Yes, the gut is a key player in immune function. A balanced gut microbiome supports immune responses, and imbalances may contribute to immune-related issues. Maintaining gut health through a nutritious diet and lifestyle practices can positively impact overall immune function.

11. Are Supplements Necessary for Gut Health?

-Answer: Supplements can be beneficial, but they should complement, not replace, a balanced diet. Probiotics, prebiotics, and certain vitamins may support gut health. Consult with healthcare professionals before incorporating supplements, as individual needs vary.

12. Can Stress Affect Gut Health?

- Answer: Yes, stress can impact gut health. **Prolonged stress may change the makeup of gut flora and aggravate digestive problems.** Practices like mindfulness, meditation, and relaxation techniques can help manage stress and support a healthy gut.

Understanding these frequently asked questions provides a foundation for making informed decisions about gut health. It highlights the interconnectedness of gut health with various aspects of well-being and encourages individuals to adopt holistic approaches for optimal digestive and overall health.

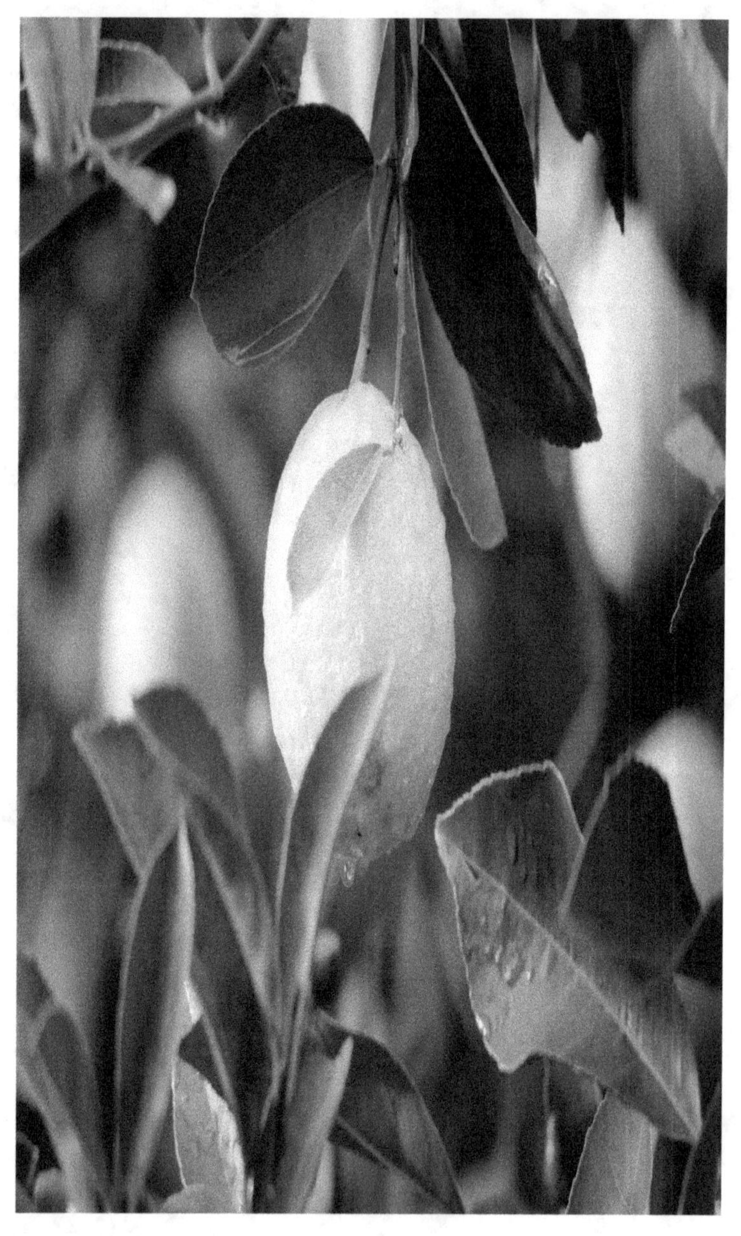

CHAPTER NINE

Understanding Gut-Boosting Supplements

1. Probiotics

-Overview: Probiotics are live beneficial bacteria that support the balance of gut microbiota. They can be found in supplements or fermented foods like yogurt, kefir, and sauerkraut.

- Benefits: Probiotics aid digestion, promote a healthy gut microbiome, and may alleviate symptoms of certain digestive disorders. Strains like Lactobacillus and Bifidobacterium are commonly used.

2. Prebiotics

-Overview: Prebiotics are non-digestible fibers that serve as food for beneficial gut bacteria. They are available as supplements and can be found in some foods..

-Benefits: Prebiotics nourish and stimulate the growth of probiotics, promoting a diverse and resilient gut microbiome. Sources include chicory root, garlic, and bananas.

3. Digestive Enzymes

-Overview: Digestive enzyme supplements contain enzymes that aid in breaking down fats, proteins, and carbohydrates. Common enzymes include amylase, protease, and lipase.

- Benefits: These supplements can enhance digestion, especially in individuals with enzyme deficiencies or conditions like pancreatic insufficiency. They may alleviate symptoms of bloating and discomfort.

4. Fish Oil (Omega-3 Fatty Acids)

-Overview:Fish oil supplements provide omega-3 fatty acids, including EPA and DHA, which have anti-inflammatory properties.

-Benefits: Omega-3s support a healthy gut lining, reduce inflammation, and contribute to a balanced gut microbiome. They may be beneficial in managing inflammatory bowel diseases.

5. Glutamine

-Overview: Glutamine is an amino acid that serves as a building block for proteins. It is available as a supplement.

-Benefits: Glutamine supports the integrity of the intestinal lining, aids in tissue repair, and may help manage conditions like leaky gut. It is crucial for maintaining a healthy gut barrier.

6. Collagen
    -Overview: Collagen supplements provide the building blocks for connective tissues, including those in the gut.
    -Benefits: Collagen supports gut health by maintaining the integrity of the intestinal lining. It may aid in conditions like leaky gut and promote overall digestive well-being.

7. Aloe Vera
    -Overview: Aloe vera supplements are derived from the inner gel of the aloe plant.
    - Benefits: Aloe vera has anti-inflammatory properties and may support digestive health. It is sometimes used to alleviate symptoms of conditions like irritable bowel syndrome (IBS).

8. Turmeric (Curcumin)
    -Overview: Turmeric supplements contain curcumin, a compound with anti-inflammatory and antioxidant properties.
    - Benefits: Curcumin may help manage inflammation in the gut, making it potentially beneficial for conditions like inflammatory bowel disease (IBD) and irritable bowel syndrome (IBS).

9. Psyllium Husk

-Overview: Psyllium husk is a soluble fiber often used as a supplement to support digestive health.

-Benefits: Psyllium husk adds bulk to stool, promotes regular bowel movements, and may help manage conditions like constipation. It acts as a prebiotic, supporting beneficial gut bacteria.

10. L-Glutathione

-Overview: L-Glutathione is an antioxidant compound naturally produced in the body. It is also available as a supplement.

-Benefits: Glutathione supports detoxification processes, reduces oxidative stress in the gut, and contributes to overall gut health.

11. Quercetin

-Overview: Quercetin is a flavonoid found in certain fruits, vegetables, and available as a supplement.

-Benefits: Quercetin has anti-inflammatory and antioxidant properties. It may help manage inflammatory conditions in the gut and support overall digestive health.

12. Deglycyrrhizinated Licorice (DGL)
   - Overview: DGL is a form of licorice where the compound glycyrrhizin, associated with potential side effects, is removed.
       -Benefits: DGL may help soothe the gastrointestinal tract, support the mucosal lining, and alleviate symptoms of conditions like acid reflux.

Considerations and Precautions
Consultation with Healthcare Professionals
   - Individuals with existing health conditions or those considering supplements should consult healthcare professionals for personalized advice.

Quality of Supplements
   - Choose reputable brands for supplements to ensure quality, purity, and accurate dosages.

Balanced Approach
   - While supplements can complement a healthy lifestyle, they should not replace a well-rounded diet rich in whole foods.

Monitoring Effects
   - Pay attention to how your body responds to supplements and adjust usage based on individual needs.

Gut-boosting supplements can play a supportive role in maintaining digestive health. However, individual responses vary, and a holistic approach that includes a nutrient-rich diet and lifestyle practices remains crucial for optimal gut well-being.

CHAPTER TEN

Sustaining a Healthy Gut for Life: A Comprehensive Guide

1. Dietary Guidelines for Gut Health

-Diverse and Fiber-Rich Foods: Prioritize a variety of colorful fruits, vegetables, whole grains, legumes, and nuts. These fiber-rich foods nourish beneficial gut bacteria.

-Probiotic-Rich Foods: Include fermented foods like yogurt, kefir, sauerkraut, and kimchi to introduce beneficial probiotics to your gut.

-Lean Proteins: Choose lean protein sources such as poultry, fish, beans, and tofu to support overall digestive health.

- Healthy Fats: Incorporate sources of healthy fats like avocados, nuts, seeds, and olive oil to promote gut well-being.

2. Hydration and Gut Health

-Adequate Water Intake: Stay well-hydrated to support digestion and maintain the mucosal lining of the intestines. Water aids in nutrient absorption and overall gut function.

-Herbal Teas: Incorporate herbal teas like peppermint or ginger, known for their digestive benefits, into your hydration routine.

3. Regular Physical Activity

-Exercise for Gut Motility: Engage in regular physical activity to stimulate the contraction of intestinal muscles, promoting the movement of food through the digestive tract.

-Moderation is Key: Strive for a balanced approach to exercise, avoiding extremes that might stress the body.

4. Prioritize Adequate Sleep

-Sleep and Gut Health: Aim for sufficient and quality sleep as it contributes to a healthy gut microbiome. Lack of sleep can impact gut bacteria balance and overall digestion.

5. Stress Management Techniques

- Mindfulness and Relaxation: Practice stress-reduction techniques such as mindfulness, meditation, deep breathing, or yoga. Gut health can be adversely affected by ongoing stress.

-Balancing Work and Relaxation: Create a balance between work and leisure to reduce stress levels and support overall well-being.

6. Avoiding Overuse of Antibiotics

-Judicious Use: Use antibiotics judiciously and only as prescribed by healthcare professionals. Excessive use can disrupt the balance of gut bacteria, leading to dysbiosis.

7. Moderate Alcohol Consumption

   - Limiting Intake: If you consume alcohol, do so in moderation. Excessive alcohol intake can negatively impact gut health, including the gut lining and microbial balance.

8. Avoiding Tobacco:

   -Quit Smoking: If you smoke, consider quitting. Smoking has adverse effects on the gut, contributing to conditions like inflammatory bowel disease (IBD) and impacting overall health.

9. Regular Health Check-ups

   -Monitoring Digestive Health: Schedule regular check-ups with healthcare professionals to address any digestive concerns promptly.

   -Screening for Conditions: Periodic screenings may be recommended, especially if there's a family history of digestive disorders.

10. Maintain a Healthy Weight

   -Balanced Nutrition and Exercise: Aim for a healthy weight through a combination of balanced nutrition and regular physical activity. Excess weight, especially around the abdominal area, can impact gut health.

11. Mindful Eating Practices

   - Chew Thoroughly: Practice mindful eating by chewing food thoroughly. This aids in the digestion process and nutrient absorption.

-Awareness of Hunger and Fullness:Pay attention to hunger and fullness cues to avoid overeating or undereating.

12. Diverse Nutrient Intake

-Incorporate Variety: Aim for a diverse nutrient intake by including a range of vitamins, minerals, and antioxidants through different food sources.

-Customized Nutrition: Consider individual dietary needs, including any specific intolerances or sensitivities, to personalize your approach.

13. Continual Learning and Adaptation

-Stay Informed: Keep abreast of new research and information related to gut health. The field is continually evolving, and staying informed empowers you to make informed choices.

-Adapt to Life Changes: Recognize that life circumstances, including age, lifestyle, and stress levels, may change. Be adaptable in your approach to sustaining gut health.

14. Seeking Professional Guidance

-Consult Healthcare Professionals: If you have specific health concerns or conditions, consult with registered dietitians, gastroenterologists, or other healthcare professionals for personalized guidance.

-Regular Check-ups: Periodic check-ups can help monitor gut health and address any emerging issues promptly.

15. Long-Term Mindset

- Consistency Over Time: Sustaining a healthy gut is a lifelong journey. Consistency in positive lifestyle choices over time is more impactful than short-term interventions.

-Celebrating Progress: Acknowledge and celebrate progress in your gut health journey, recognizing that small, consistent efforts yield long-term benefits.

Sustaining a healthy gut for life involves a holistic and mindful approach to nutrition, lifestyle, and overall well-being. By incorporating these comprehensive strategies into your daily life, you can support a resilient gut and promote optimal digestive health throughout the various stages of life. Remember, it's a journey, and each positive choice contributes to your long-term well-being.

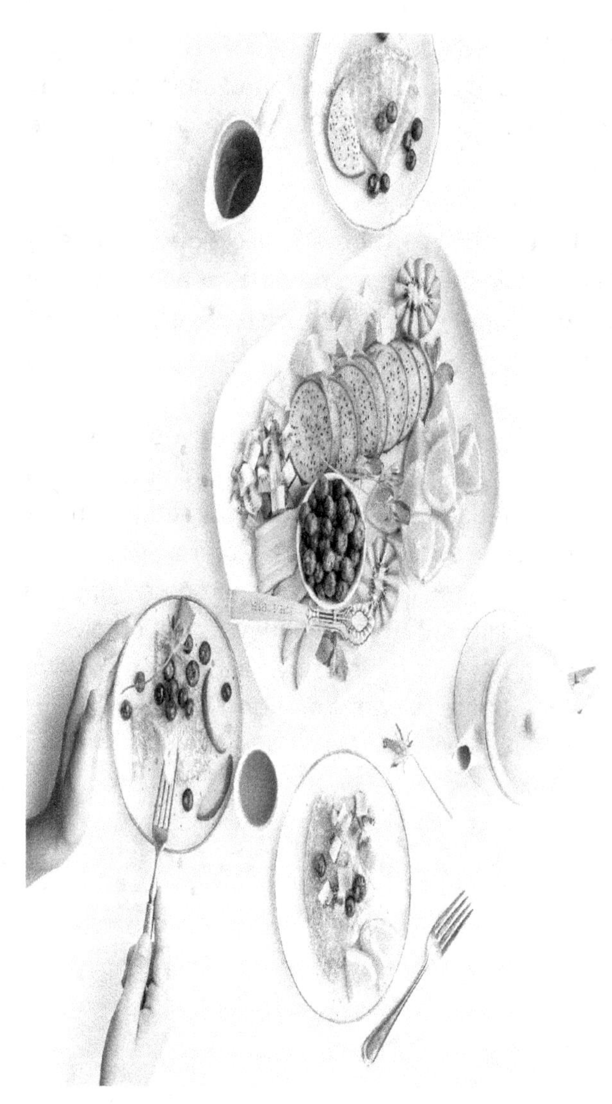

CONCLUSION

As we conclude our journey through "The Healthy Gut Diet Book," it's evident that fostering gut health is not just a fleeting trend but a commitment to a lifelong partnership with our bodies. This comprehensive guide has delved into the intricate world of the gut, offering insights, practical tips, and a wealth of knowledge to empower you on your path to digestive vitality.

From understanding the foundations of gut health to exploring the key components of a nourishing diet, this book has aimed to equip you with the tools needed to make informed choices. We've discussed the significance of diverse nutrients, the benefits of mindful eating, and the impact of lifestyle on our gut microbiome.

Meal planning, recipes, and dietary recommendations have been laid out with the intention of inspiring not just temporary changes, but sustainable habits that resonate with your unique lifestyle. Whether you're preparing gut-friendly breakfasts to kickstart your day or savoring savory lunch and dinner options, each recipe is crafted to harmonize flavor with gut-loving ingredients.

Our exploration of gut-boosting supplements and lifestyle tips has emphasized that maintaining gut health is a holistic endeavor. It encompasses not only what we eat but how we live – from managing stress to getting quality sleep and engaging in regular physical activity.

In the realm of gut-friendly recipes and mindful snacking, we've celebrated the diversity of flavors and textures that contribute not only to our pleasure in eating but also to the flourishing of our gut microbiome. The benefits of lean proteins, whole grains, and plant-based foods in promoting gut health have been highlighted, emphasizing a balanced and varied approach to nourishing our bodies.

As we navigate the frequently asked questions surrounding gut health and dispel common misconceptions, we recognize the importance of informed choices. The journey to sustaining a healthy gut is personalized, acknowledging that individual needs, preferences, and responses vary.

In the chapter on gut-boosting supplements, we've explored additional tools to support digestive well-being. However, the overarching theme remains clear – supplements complement, but they do not replace the foundation of a nutrient-rich diet and a lifestyle that prioritizes the health of our gut.

The guide concludes by addressing the lifelong commitment to gut well-being. It goes beyond a book's final pages, urging you to integrate the principles shared here into your daily existence. By incorporating diverse nutrients, practicing mindfulness, and seeking balance in all aspects of life, you embark on a journey that extends far beyond a singular dietary regimen.

In essence, "The Healthy Gut Diet Book" is an invitation to a lifetime of digestive vitality. It's a roadmap that encourages you to savor the joys of eating, embrace the wisdom of nourishing your body, and celebrate the symbiotic relationship between what you consume and how you thrive. May your journey towards a healthy gut be filled with flavor, joy, and the sustained well-being that comes from nurturing yourself from the inside out.

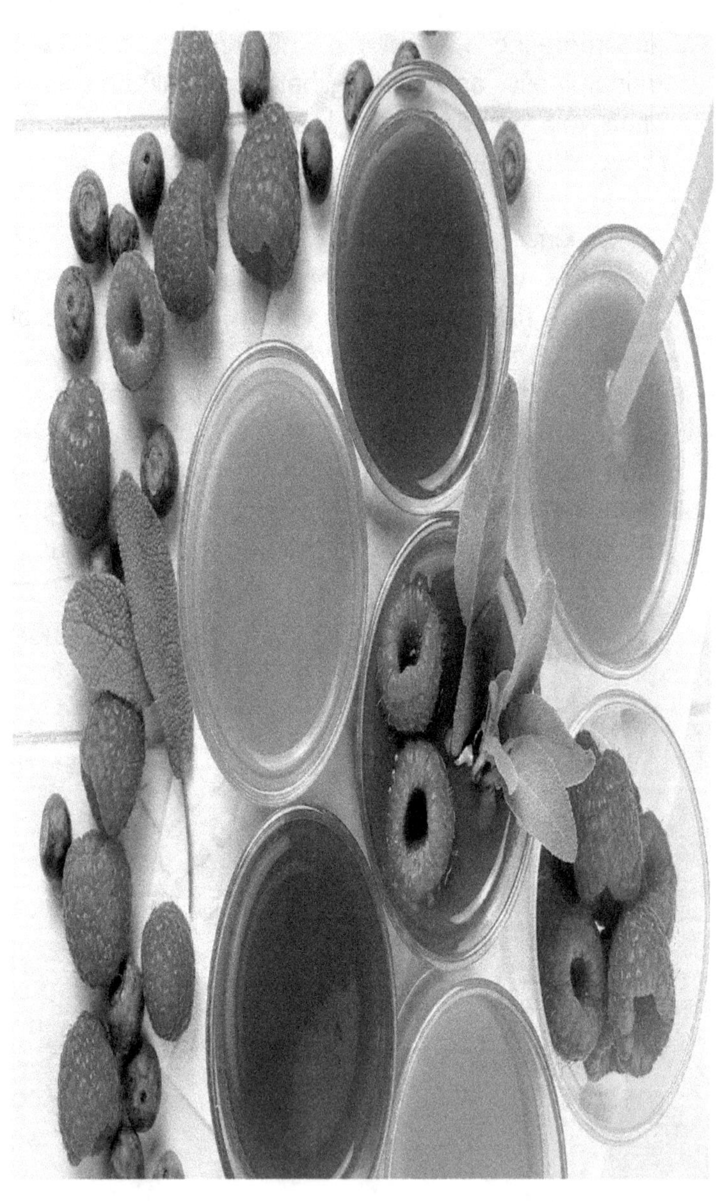

www.ingramcontent.com/pod-product-compliance
Lightning Source LLC
Chambersburg PA
CBHW061002260726
48661CB00005B/2015